CONTENTS

FIt Diary Volume 2

By Rita Ferdinando

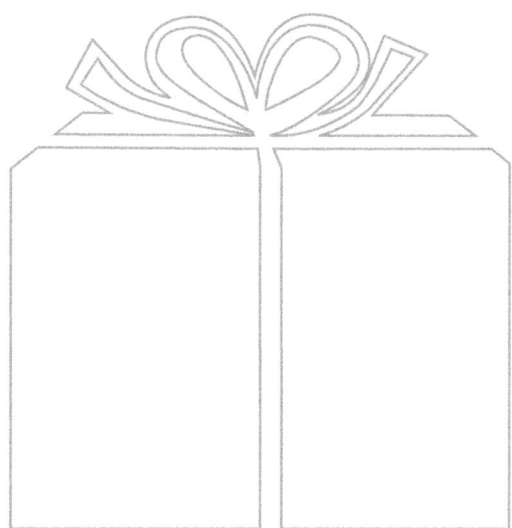

A c k n o w l e d g e m e n t s : *This Book Was Written So That You Will Have The Motivation To Eat Healthy!*

Fit Diary
Volume 2
Remember To Change Your Routine!

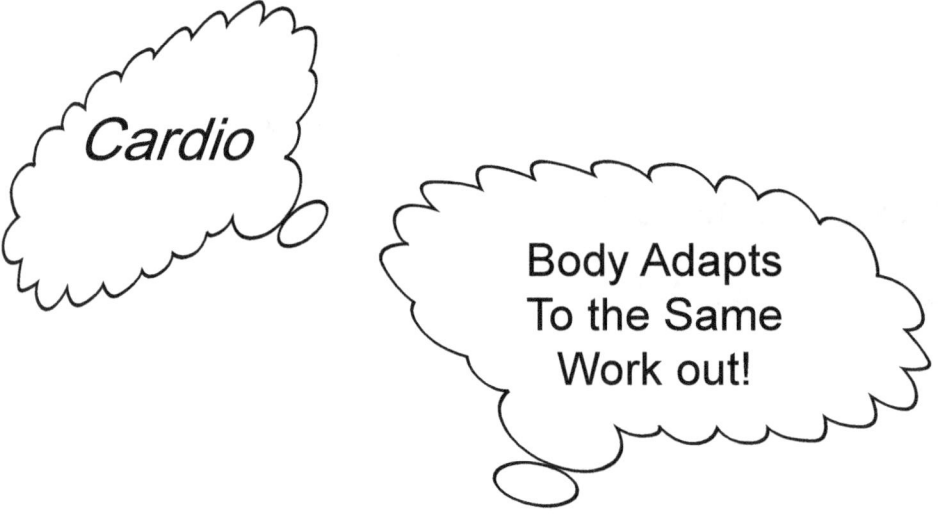

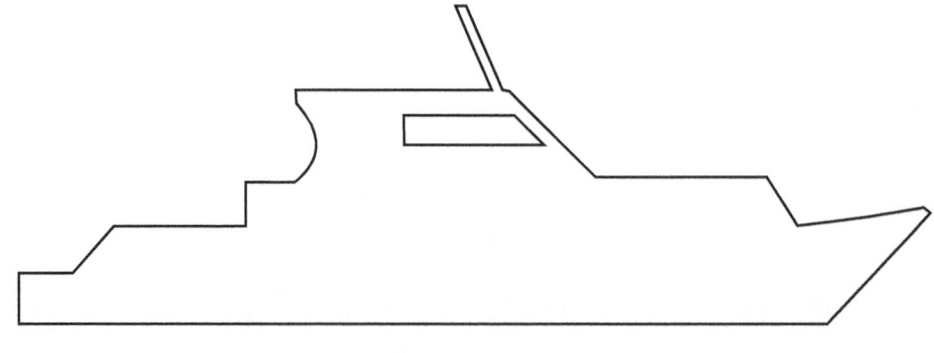

Your Notes

Fit Diary
Lifting

More Reps
Or 8 - 12

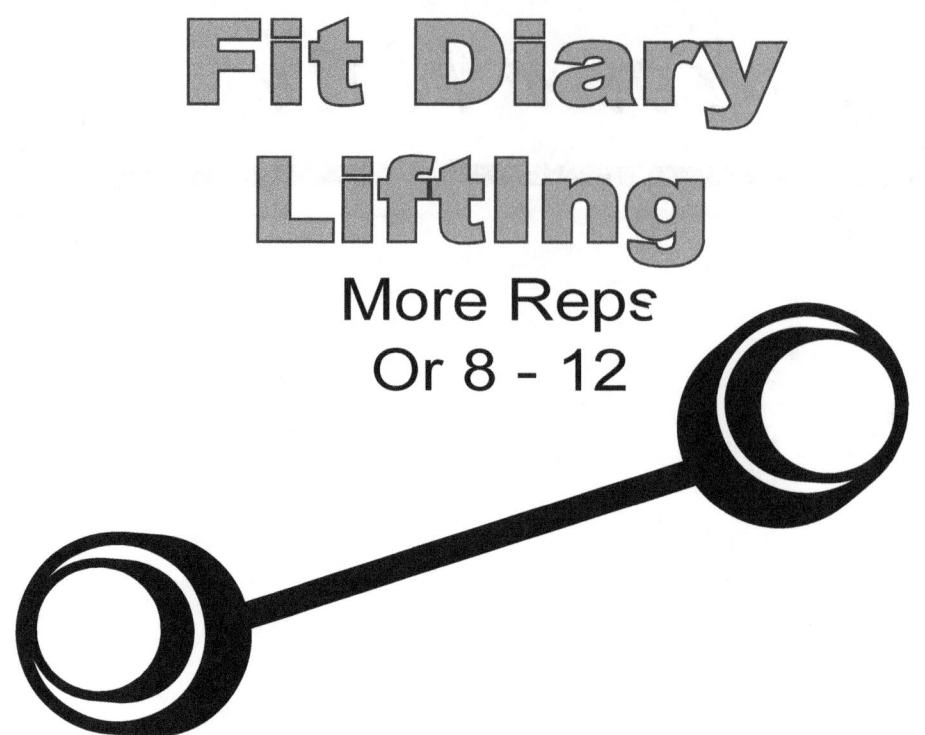

Your Notes

Your Notes

Cardio

Cardio

Your Notes

Eating Better

What To Eat?

Monday
Tuesday
Wednesday
Thursday
Friday
Saturday Day
Sunday

What Are You Eating?

Your Notes

Breakfast ?

Your Notes

Your Notes

Breakfast

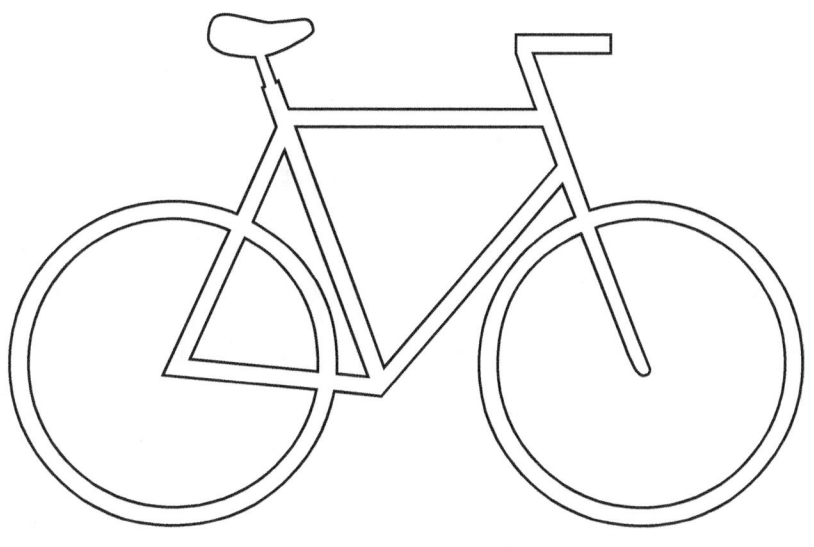

Lunch ?

Your Notes

Lunch

Your Notes

Dinner ?

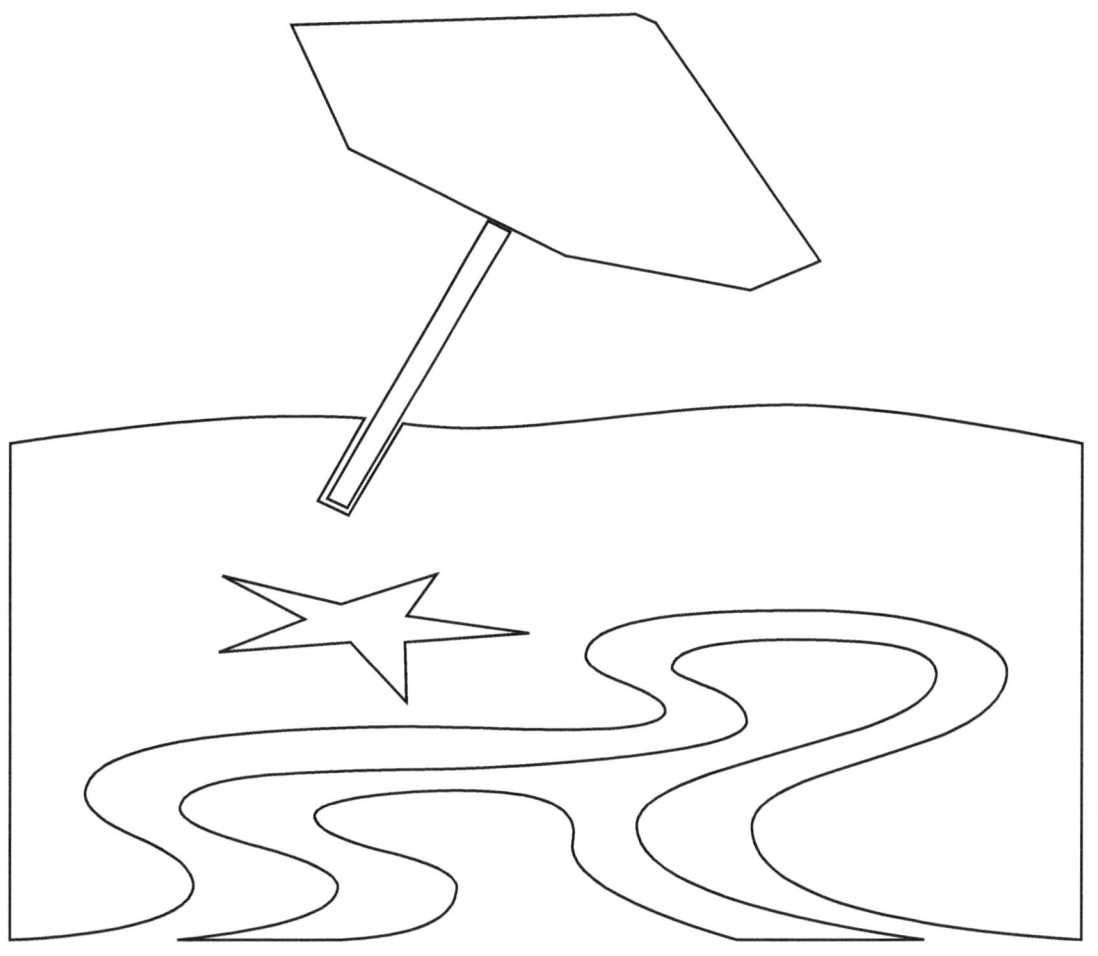

Your Notes

Dinner ?

Your Notes

Lite Exercise

Your Notes

Snacks

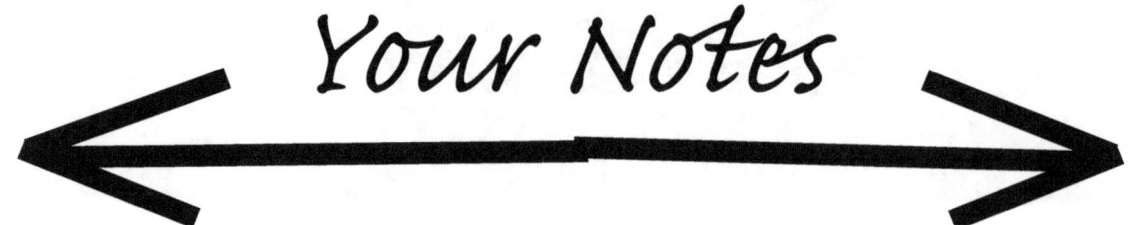

Your Notes

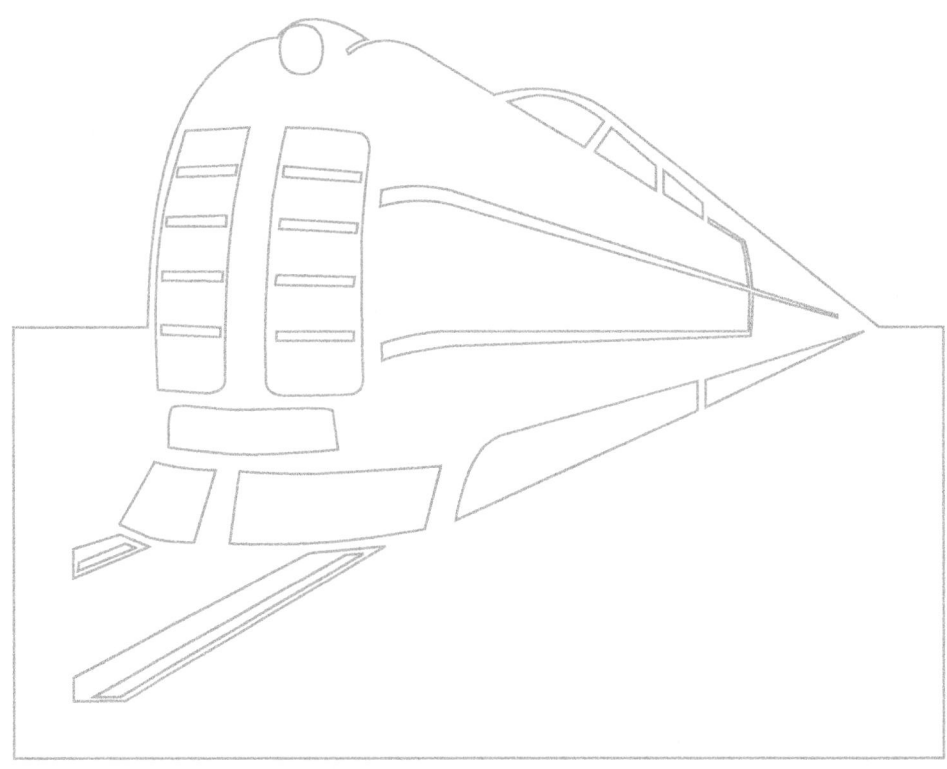

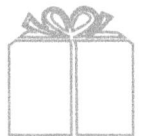 This Book Was Written So That You Will
Have The Motivation To Eat Healthy And Change Your Routine!
Book Design by Author Rita Ferdinando